THE NAKED TRUTH ABOUT HOLISTIC HEALTH

THE NAKED TRUTH ABOUT HOLISTIC HEALTH

Nemmsaiu Amen-Sebek, N.D.

Copyright © 2010 by Nemmsaiu Amen-Sebek, N.D.

Library of Congress Control Number:		2010907395
ISBN:	Hardcover	978-1-4535-0842-8
	Softcover	978-1-4535-0841-1
	Ebook	978-1-4535-0843-5

This book was printed in the United States of America.

To order additional copies of this book, contact:
Xlibris Corporation
1-888-795-4274
www.Xlibris.com
Orders@Xlibris.com
81650

CONTENTS

TRUTH ABOUT NATURE'S HERBS

Everything you put into your mouth affects your body. Everything you put on your skin enters your blood, everything you smell, you have breathed as well as tasted.

Herbs are Nature's medicine chest. Nature is called the Neteru.

The key to using herbs is not the remedies, but an understanding in herbal actions. The principle of using these herbs is based upon holistic healing, which means, spirit, mind and body. There is medical healing and emotional healing, the herbs will deal with both, but the healer needs to beware of which direction they are assisting the client.

The environmental factors of today, have put all of life in some un-natural stress situations. The government has forsaken the people, and sold the food to chemist (factories). Our health is now based on being sick, and the medicines aren't designed to cure. The prescribed drugs sold to us through the doctors and by the pharmacist is nothing more than approved laboratory testing on the population at large, just to make another billion dollars or two, which is why the medical field is called a "practice" and guess who they get to practice on, and you pay for it, in more ways than money.

American medicine has a barbaric history, with Barbers being the first doctors, using a technique called "blood letting". This was called surgery. Gyn/Ob was founded at the expense of Afrakan slave women subjected to inhumane techniques which was nothing less than torture, by Dr. Marion Simms, during the 1800's. American medicine is also younger than all other kultures, Americans also have the most diseases, and the most unhealthy people than any other kulture, and Americans also own more patents on deadly human viruses than any other kulture. We have a sick kulture that continues to practice medicine from a sick point of view.

You must practice healthy activities to have a healthy life. These activities consist of your lifestyle, which covers your whole being, spiritually, mentally, and physically, and you should look at yourself as nothing less than that, or you will be healing yourself from a segmented point of view, which isn't holistic or natural. The whole being is how one thinks, how one eats, how one connects to God, how one has sex, etc.

Tai chi and yoga are considered holistic forms of exercising.

Nature or the Neteru is the Creator doing things according to the natural order of things, and there we find the methods of restoring ourselves back to a healthy state of being. That which is un-natural (prescribed medicines) can not cure that which is natural (heaven created man/woman). We live in a time when wealth is all supreme, even at the expense of health, so the hospitals have gone into the economic business, and they experiment with health.

What makes this very serious is that allopathic medicine has lost sight of what good health truly is. We have been tricked, hoodwinked, and bamboozled.

The numbers used to measure our health is a language, but allopathic medicine still being in its infant but deadly stages, has yet to learn how to apply this language correctly, so that a better understanding of health is achieved by the population. Drs. Have learned how to scare their patients with the language they use, so it isn't a user friendly type of communication, and should be.

So let us embark on this journey back to nature, where we will find our true selves and restore our health, not just to ourselves, but to earth, mother earth.

EATING

Our eating habits and our lifestyles are the determining factor of the level of our health. Correct eating will prevent bad health, and restore good health. To be healthy is a birthright, but we have been tricked, bamboozled, and hoodwinked about what good health is, nothing out weighs the dollar including human life, in America.

Maat Principles of eating

Truth—am I really hungry, am I feeding my emotion or my body?
Justice—Does my choice of food give nutritional justice to my body?
Righteousness—Is the food good for God's temple?
Harmony—How does junk food balance with my body?
Order—Does the food follow the correct order?
Propriety—Is the food adding to my wellness, and helping me to eliminate?
Compassion—Do I accept that my wellness adds to the benefit of my culture?
Reciprocity—Am I using food to commit suicide, to punish myself?

We must learn to eat according to our life style for that day, as the animals do in Nature.

WHAT MAKES THE HERB?

The main parts of the plant are the root, stem, flower (fruit/seeds), and or leaf. Different parts of the plant can be used to focus on specific parts of the body, for example: the root will be rich in minerals; the stem will be good for circulation and the fruit rich in vitamins and minerals. There is a concept called the *"Doctrine of Signatures"* which is an Afrakan concept describing how to recognize the usage of herbs according the environment they are growing, whether the leaves are smooth or wrinkled, the color of the fruit, as well as shape and taste. If the leaf is wrinkled it is usually good for the skin, if smooth then it is good for smooth organs. If one color then generally used for one organ. The environment, if it grows high in the mountains, then it is usually good for the respiratory system, if near water then usually good for the circulatory system. Sweet taste, then high in minerals. It is important to remember that the list is more extensive than this, and all the categories should be used to conjunction with each other, when using the concept. There are herbs that are poisonous to humans and not to animals, so beware. In some instances you can watch which plants the animals eat to know which one is safe. Sometimes the antidote to the poisonous plant will be growing in the immediate area, and the combination of the two could be a medical formula.

Unless you are packing your own herbs, the products will already come packaged in accordance with which part of the plant should be used. Therefore your main concern will be the amount and which herbs work best together. Most herbs have multiple uses, but as you become comfortable with using them you will recognize their primary usage, which is important when combining herbs. Directions will come with the products, follow the directions unless you are deep into the disharmony, then you can double the dosage for approximately a week, and then return back to the recommended dosage. You should consult a holistic healer with any concerns of using specific dosages.

DOCTRINE OF SIGNATURES

Herbs that grow in a specific area will usually contain properties to keep one healthy that lives in that same area. Mountains herbs are good for lungs, bruises, stabilization of temperature, resistance to cold, and blood pressure regulation. Herbs in water, control fluid absorption, resistance to circulatory illness, aid the internal nerves and blood system or organs, diuretic properties. 90% of herbs that grow in water are edible. Herbs that grow in the desert aid electrolyte balance, regulate water in the body, hold moisture in the skin, stabilize the temperature, help heal burns, and can protect you from ultra violet rays. Herbs that grow near water, hair, skin, lung dis-eases, dissolve waste and aid in the retention of oils in the body.

A Leaf with many veins is good for circulation, straight veins or have no vein branches attached to the main vein's trunk are good for muscles. Complex vein formations are for nerve and circulatory diseases. Simple formations are good for muscles, digestive tissues and bones. Leaves that shine have high content of oil. Leaves that have the shape of an organ are good for that organ. Use color chart, and vein shapes of the eye chart.

Taste, bitter, is astringent, and may be alkaline. Sweet, high in minerals, this herb can open up pores. Diaphoretic.

Colors, Red fruit roots are good for blood disease, circulatory system.
Yellow fruit roots are good for bowel disease, diabetes
Brown root with inner yellow flesh is good for intestinal disease.
Brown root with soft inner flesh and white color is good for hollow organs (Intestines, bladder, stomach)
Brown root with hard inner white flesh is good for solid organs (kidneys, heart, and liver)

Fruit herbs with thorns are generally edible. The skin of the fruit changes color, then edible. Fruit skin that can be peeled, usually high in mineral content. Use color chart.

PAIN KILLERS

Pain killers are the most abused drug used. They are extremely destructive to the liver, mainly aspirins, especially one that begins with a T.

Pain mustn't be approached from the point of view of just getting rid of it, but what is causing it. Pain is a signal, a signal of distress. Help is being called for. Sometimes the body has the necessary ability to relieve the pain, and sometimes it requires some assistance. The body only understands one thing, and that is how to live, therefore it is going to do whatever it needs for survival of the whole.

Allopathic medicine will suppress the pain, which isn't a cure. The problem still exists and without proper attention it will eventually get worse. Allopathic medicine will prohibit, which is the act of shutting down the functioning of some normal activity in the body, which becomes dangerous when the body is in need of that activity. Once again that is not a cure. The Creator has provided all that man needs, which is written in many so-called holy books, but seldom exercised, or discussed by the people reading those books. Man can not improve on God(dess), yet we continue to fool ourselves and call it technology, which we have no idea of what the word represents. It stands for all things not natural, because nature is the only true technology, and that came from the heaven, and if there is nothing greater than God(dess), then there can be no greater gift than that which comes from heaven.

Let us explore some natural (nature's herbs) pain killers and how to use them.

The most common is **white willow:** it is a nerve sedative, it works like an aspirin except it is mild on the stomach, and it has strong benign antiseptic abilities for infected wounds and isn't harmful to the liver.

Valerian: it relaxes muscle spasms, and has pain relieving properties, can be used with white willow. It is recommended for short term usage. It is rich in magnesium, potassium and zinc.

Catnip: is nature's "alka seltzer", it has a sedative effect on the nervous system, helps to induce sleep, and perspiration without heating the body. Good for flu and fevers. It contains magnesium, manganese, vitamin A & C, and B complex.

Chamomile: good for soothing stomach ailments, especially for children. It soothes the nerves and menstrual cramps. It is high in calcium, magnesium and potassium. Also helps with mental alertness in children.

Feverfew: good for migraines, no side effects.

Lemon grass: good for people under stress and women suffering from cramps, headaches and dizziness. High in vitamin A & C.

Mullein: has narcotic properties, but not habit forming. A great pain killer, and induces sleep. Great for coughs and colds, it loosens mucus. It helps with sore throats and high in iron.

Some other interesting facts about using pain killers, the un-natural ones, whether they be over the counter, or prescribed:

Just one normal dose of aspirin, can reduce your melatonin by 75%.
Aspirin also blocks the absorption of Vitamin C, and folic acid
One of the most common types of pain is arthritis. Osteoarthritis is the most common form, and affects women more than men. Most women are calcium deficient. That is why they have a higher rate of osteoarthritis. Vitamin C helps with the absorption of iron, which is connected to calcium.
For women hormone imbalance is a cause of headaches. Lack of progesterone, and excess of estrogen.
When an excess of estrogen is present, salt and fluid retention may occur, which interferes with thyroid hormone, reducing the level of oxygen in cells, and reducing vascular tone.

There are other pain relieving herbs, such as arnica which works well topically. For stomach problems you can look right in your kitchen. A kitchen herb like Turmeric/curcumin is a powerful anti-inflammatory, and a natural cortisone. Garlic is good for the overall immune system.

Remember that all drugs are hard on the body, and they will do damage to the Liver, because everything is processed through the Liver. The Liver must be given some help in restoring its self, it is the only organ in the body that can repair a majority of its self. Unfortunately is it not designed to handle the break-down of the drugs and chemicals given to us through the Allopathic world and food.

Two herbs we must keep in mind are **Dandelion** and **Milk thistle** to keep the Liver healthy; these herbs can be safely taken with the herbs mentioned earlier for pain.

Anytime one gets involved in taking drugs (prescribed medicine), it will produce high toxicity, and the liver will have to be de-toxed, to help it back to health. Never forget nutrition as part of your healing, the rawer the food the healthier it will be for the body and the proper nutrients will be absorbed.

ANTI-BIOTICS

The anti-biotics used by the medical profession are truly killing the world, they are the cause of some of the worse viruses and bacteria on the planet and these antibiotics are being distributed by the hospitals, the same place that is supposedly helping our health, has created real entities that are killing our health.

Antibiotics activate a higher intelligence within the bacteria, which allows them to turn into what we know as "Super Bugs"

The belief or era of "Miracle drugs" has long ended. Penicillin was created in 1928, it became a routine use. Although the doctor who created it, Dr. Flemming, warned that forms of bacteria were already becoming resistant to it, and by 1945 it would be of little effect. By 1950, 59% was resistant to it. A new generation of bacteria is produced every twenty two (22) minutes.

Let us examine some natural ways through Nature (Neteru), in dealing with these harmful bacteria and viruses, with the usage of herbs:

Acacia—*primarily found in Afraka & Asia—active against Stapylococcus, aureus, malaria, salmonella, and shigella dysenteriae.*

Aloe—*active against herpes simplex, Staphylococcus aureus. To be used externally. It also has antibacterial properties. Used with honey, it is good to close up open wounds.*

Echinacea—*good against bacterial and viral infections. May be used for an infection anywhere in the body. Used with Yarrow or Bearberrry, it effectively stops cystitis. Anti-microbial.*

Garlic—*has universal usage. For the digestive tract garlic will support the development of the natural bacterial flora. It reduces blood pressure. Anit-microbial. It is also an antiseptic, and anti-spasmodic.*

Ginger—*one of its clinical uses is for burns, juice of fresh ginger, soaked into a cotton ball and applied to burns, acts as an immediate pain reliever. Also good for malaria.*

Licorice—*an immune system stimulus. Antibacterial activity, also a catalyst for other herbs.*

Wormwood—*good for sore infections in the throat and lungs. It numbs the pain. Effective against malaria.*

What makes herbs more effective against bacteria and viruses is the fact that they contain dozen of compounds, which overwhelms the bacteria and viruses, before they can develop resistance to it. Once one knows how to use the herbs, the combinations become extremely effective, although herbs work slowly as they help to restore the body. Remember the key to restoring harmony is the ability to mix the correct combinations of herbs.

Now allow us to look at the categories of herbs, to get a better understanding of their primary properties, for the purpose of recognizing what combinations should be considered for specific harmonies.

THE ACTION OF HERBS

Listed below are various categories of herbs, what their properties are, and of course the list can be expanded, but we have listed some of the more common as well as the best for the job. We only list some of the more common categories.

Alterative—these herbs gradually restore the proper function of the body and increase health and vitality. They have also been known as "blood cleansers" *burdock, cleavers, Echinacea, red clover, garlic, golden seal, sarsaparilla, wild indigo, yellow dock.*

Anti-catarrhal—these herbs help to remove excess toxinsfrom the body, catarrhal build-ups. *Boneset, golden rod, mullein, sage, marshmallow, coltsfoot.*

Anti-inflammatory—these herbs combat inflammation. *Devils claw, marigold, witch hazel, chamomile, feverfew, cat's claw, arnica.*

Anti-microbial—these are infection herbs, they help to destroy pathogens. *Echinacea, garlic, juniper, thyme, marigold, wild indigo.*

Anti-spasmodic—these herbs help prevent spasms and cramps. *Black cohosh, chamomile, cramp bark, lobelia, valerian, wild lettuce, skullcap, motherwort.*

Astringent—these herbs contract tissue. *Agrimony, bayberry, slippery elm, witch hazel, shepards purse.*

Cardiac Toners—herbs that affect the heart. *Hawthorn, motherwort.*

Calmatives—valerian, hops, catnip, skullcap, passion flower.

Demulcent—*these herbs soothe and protect irritated or inflamed internal tissue. Coltsfoot, comfrey, irish moss, marshmallow, slippery elm.*

Diaphoretic—*perspiration, and elimination of toxins in the skin.* ***Pleurisy root, angelica, buchu, cayenne, garlic, yarrow.***

Diuretic—increases the secretion and elimination of urine. ***Buchu, corn silk, dandelion, juniper.***

Expectorant—these herbs support the body in removing mucus from the respiratory system. ***Pleurisy, chickweed, comfrey, elecampane, skunk cabbage.***

Stimulants—these herbs excite the body. Stimulant herbs are required in smaller doses to excite the body. ***Cayenne, yellow root, cinnamon, ginseng, yohimbe, cloves.***

Now that we have some idea of how herbs work, and their properties, we can start to put our formulas together. The study of vitamins is also very helpful in utilizing these formulas; we won't spend much time talking about the properties of the vitamins, but may include some in the formulas as well as minerals.

These formulas are just suggested recommendations. A holistic healer should be consulted.

DISHARMONIES & THEIR SINGLE NATURAL REMEDIES

In many cases you will only need to mix 3 to 4 herbs together to get desired results. Monitor the disharmony every 2-4 weeks, after 30 days you may want to change up the formula or take a week break from using the herbs.

Some herbs are more potent than others, even though they don't have any harmful side effects, can develop a dependency.

Abcess: an accumulation of pus, inflammation and tenderness. This is a skin disorder, therefore a formula may include: *Burdock, dandelion root, Echinacea, red clover, garlic, myrrh.*

Acne: skin inflammation: *cleavers, burdock, wild indigo, marigold, blue flag.*

Arthritis: is first a symptom, the body is filling up with toxic waste, which is crystallizing in the joints: *corn silk, devil's claw, silver burch, yarrow, bladderwack, burdock, white willow bark, licorice root.*

Blood Pressure (high): *hawthorn, garlic, celery, ginkgo biloba, kelp, motherwort.*

Bruises: bruises bring pain, and inflammation: *Arnica, marigold, calendula, chickweed, St. John's wort.*

Burns: burns are cooked tissue, 1st degree being just the outer skin, to 3rd degree burns, where muscle, nerves and tissues are cooked, this being the worse: *aloe, chickweed, burdock, white willow, St. John's wort.*

Colds: colds are the body trying to fight off some type of infection, so you don't catch a cold, you develop one. It causes a mucus build up: *elderberries, garlic, Echinacea, golden seal, catnip, slippery elm, rose hips.*

Constipation: keep in mind it takes 4 hours for the stomach to empty: *buckthorn, cascara sagrada, rhubarb root, senna, black root, flax seed.*

Eczema: skin problem with rashes: *burdock, nettles, yellow dock, primrose, chickweed.*

Fever: a fever is the body trying to rid its self of a disharmony, which is a cleansing process: *boneset, catnip, ginger, peppermint, chamomile.*

Hay fever: exposure to an allergen: *ephedra,(combine nettle & licorice), also the combination of black cohosh, skullcap, pleurisy root, catnip, and red pepper.*

Headaches: headaches are usually the body sending a signal that something is wrong. Therefore the are variety of ways of approaching headaches, some come from stress, some the environment, some from the foods we eat, and some because various parts of the body are beginning to shut down, so if these combinations don't work, then the person will need a complete analysis: *feverfew, rosemary, skullcap, chamomile, St. John's wort, marjoram, wood betony.*

Hypertension: you can use the same herbs you would for high blood pressure, along with the ones listed: *butcher's broom, cayenne, garlic, hawthorn berry, rosemary.*

Indigestion: Use the herbs for constipation along with: *fennel, peppermint, valerian, wild yam, wormwood.*

Infections: use the antibiotic herbs

Kidney stones: this is crystallized waste, that the kidney can't break down: *cornsilk, couchgrass, gravel root, gingko, juniper berries, lobelia, bearberry.*

Menstruation (excessive): this is generally from a poor diet: *periwinkle, lady's mantle, blue cohosh, red raspberry, false unicorn.* If painful add *cramp bark, Jamaican dogwood, valerian, wild lettuce, chaste tea.*

Migraine: *feverfew, kola, Jamaican dogwood, peppermint, skullcap.*

Milk stimulation: *milk thistle, borage, fennel, fenugreek.*

Pain: *black cohosh, Jamaican dogwood, valerian, white willow, hops.*

Prostate: *horsetail, saw palmetto, corn silk, damiana, couchgrass.*

Sciatica: *black cohosh, Jamaican dogwood, st. john's wort.*

Toothache: *put clove oil on the tooth, just a small amount.*

Varicose veins: *shepards purse, horse chestnut, witch hazel, wild alum root.*

Water retention: *cornsilk, buchu, juniper berry, dandelion, uva ursi, horsetail.*

Vitamin A can be added when repairing tissue, or promoting the growth of new tissue. Vitamin B6 & B12 to be added for digestion problems. Vitamin C can always be added, but it is a good antioxidant. Use Zinc whenever you are trying to heal the body.

Warning whenever surgery is scheduled, the usage of these herbs and vitamins must be curtailed. They can make the medicine less effective which means they will have to give you larger doses, or make the medicine too effective, and your body may over re-act. Consult a Holistic Health professional.

BODY TONICS

Body tonics are herbs which are specifically designed to strengthen certain parts of the body;

Infections—*garlic, Echinacea, golden seal, aloe, usnea.*

Cardiovascular—*hawthorn, garlic, motherwort. Buckwheat and lime blossom are effective in strengthening blood vessels.*

Respiratory system—*mullein, elecampane, and coltsfoot.*

Digestive system—*bitter herbs are helpful, dandelion root, gentian & agrimony.*

The Liver—*milk thistle and bitter herbs*

Urinary system—*buchu, bearberry, cornsilk. (burning sensation use couchgrass)*

Reproductive system—*for women use false unicorn and raspberry, for men, saw palmetto, damiana, sarsaparilla.*

Nervous system—*oats, skullcap, St. John's wort, vervain, mugworts, ginseng.*

Musculo/skeletal system—*celery seed, nettles,(comfrey and horsetail will strengthen bones)*

The skin—*cleavers, nettles, burdock and red clovers.*

Now that we have looked at various herbs, their properties, and what disharmonies they work best on, let us now discover how the body operates and reacts. We shall briefly discuss some of the body's systems.

There is a critical acid/alkaline balance inside of the body, that varies according the needs of the body. But it must never become to excessive one way or the other. Alkalinity can kill you just as acidity can. People who are on a meat diet, without question have accumulated an acidic body, fore all animal products are acid. The liver must process everything that comes into the body, and it isn't designed to handle these acid foods. Sadly many of the foods are synthetic, especially since the FDA has approved the sale of clone meat to the public.

The colon is the key to good health. Inside of the colon, nutrients and water are absorbed back into the body. If the colon is covered with plaque, and the walls are weak, then the absorption is minimal at best, that is unhealthy. Sugar is the number one addictive drug in the world. Therefore most of us are sugar addicts and/or salt addicts, because sugar and salt are put into almost all foods. These processed additives are poisons.

THE BODY'S SYSTEMS

(how the body works)

The nervous system; comprised of the brain, spinal cord, nerves and all the chemical messengers that ensure communication throughout the body systems. The brain and the nerves speak to each other, as does each individual cell, through a group of chemicals called neurotransmitters.

Three separate systems; central nervous system (cns), this is the brain and spinal cord. Autonomic nervous system (ans), this controls involuntary functions such as heart rate, digestion, and glandular function. Peripheral nervous system (pns), this connects the (cns) to all the body tissues and voluntary muscles.

The musculoskeletal system, consist of the bones, joints, muscles and connective tissue. When musculoskeletal misalignments occur we become prone to a wide range of health problems. Everyone carries some degree of stress in their muscles. If that stress is prolonged, it can lead to chronically contracted muscles which cause the underlying structure of the body to pull and contract. The musculoskeletal system has a cause and effect relationship with the entire body. Improper body alignment can impede blood flow.

The immune system, is a complex network of organs, cells, and substances. The organs from different systems contribute to this system. This system is the primary defense against disharmonies, and pathogens. The first line of defense is the skin and gastrointestinal tract. The second line of defense is the bloodstream and the inflammatory process. The third line of defense is the involvement of organs, such as the spleen, liver, and lymph nodes.

The Lymphatic system is a subset to the immune system and acts as the body's "master drain." The lymph flows slowly through the body to the thoracic duct; body movement helps this system function. The thoracic duct drains into the bloodstream, and the toxins are transported to the liver and kidney where they are broken down and excreted.

The Endocrine system is comprised of the pineal, pituitary, hypothalamus, thyroid, adrenals, pancreas, sex glands, lungs, heart. These glands release hormones directly into the bloodstream to maintain balance and harmony within the body. This is a sensitive messenger service between the higher brain glands, and their end organ glands.

The Respiratory system is comprised of the nose, larynx, trachea, bronchi and the lungs. This system provides oxygen to every cell in the body while also expelling carbon dioxide. During cellular respiration glucose and other small molecules are oxidized to produce energy.

Organs

Each organ has a complimentary organ. When one is trying to heal or be healed the complimentary organ must be taken into consideration.

Lungs—large intestines
Heart—small intestines
Kidneys—bladder (sex organs)
Spleen—stomach
Liver—gall bladder

You also have an organ clock to be aware of, as well as a body cycle, which is physical days and mental days.

Unfortunately we are on man's clock which is out of balance with Nature's clock. So we are on a cycle other than the one to be healthy humans. We eat during the wrong hours, we have sex at the wrong hours, we study sciences at the wrong hour. With all this wrong going on, how can we be right! The Creators forgiveness lays in Nature for us all.

FORMULAS

We are now going to look at how to put a formula together. Keeping in mind an experienced natural healer will know how to add vitamins, minerals and foods to these formulas, when needed, we will only look at the herbal formulas, and how to put them together. Listed are a few disharmonies to illustrate.

Let's start with **Acne**, which is a skin disharmony. It is constipation in the skin; the skin is trying to release toxins, that weren't eliminated through your bowels. *Skin herbs: burdock, chickweed removal of toxins: Shepard's purse, Echinacea, garlic. Aloe is an antibiotic that can be used topically, so my formula would be: burdock, Echinacea, garlic, and topically some aloe. Witch hazel is an astringent, which could also be used. There is a difference between the witch hazel herb and the alcohol witch hazel in the drug store. You could also add some cleavers. The herbs can be mixed in equal parts, two or three cups a day, and cut back on fried foods.*

Allergies: allergic reactions are multiplying, manifesting themselves not only as common symptoms of sneezing, headaches and rashes, but also as changes in personality and emotions. In most allergic reactions, the immune system mis-identifies a substance as an invader. This is called auto-immune, the body starts to attack itself. Common responses to this are asthma, eczema, hay fever or headaches. Allergies are an over-reaction usually affecting the respiratory system; *fenugreek, marshmallow, pleurisy root, chaparral.* The adrenal glands must be addressed. They produce hormones: *astragalus, licorice root.* Some decongestant herbs: *ginger root, fennel seed, also something for the blood.* A general formula may look like: *Marshmallow root, burdock, mullein, astragalus, echinacea if I need it stronger add some capsicum (cayenne).*

Blood pressure: Blood pressure medicine is a big seller in the pharmaceutical world, and a big killer, to the unaware. Your blood pressure changes throughout the day as it should, when you are active, it will increase, if you have eaten the wrong foods, or had a smoke, it can increase, and if you are medications, that could keep it increased. Therefore, you should take several readings during the day to find an average of what your B/P is.

This is a heart and artery problem, not a cholesterol problem. The number one cause of a poor heart is nutrition deficiency. The arteries become weak because of this, and become blocked because of junk from poor eating. Cholesterol helps to repair arterial walls. *A formula might look like this: Hawthorn, garlic, cayenne, Siberian ginseng, motherwort and some magnesium.(magnesium is a mineral).* If one is having palpations, then the formula changes slightly, but you can't go wrong with *Hawthorn, garlic and magnesium, add valerian or passion flower for the palpations.*

Colds: You don't catch a cold, no more than you can catch good health, it is the manifestation of an infection in your body, the cold is showing it to you. The cold is actually a cleansing process trying to rid itself of the infection. We are dealing with an immune problem, which means strengthening the blood, the liver, and the colon. Some of the signs are a cough, which means the lungs or respiratory system, it could include a headache, which means using herbs like: *gingko biloba, white willow, and feverfew.* A formula: *goldenseal, garlic, mullein, coltsfoot, slippery elm, and maybe some comfrey.*

Cholesterol: This one the doctors have done an outstanding job in tricking the people. High cholesterol is a symptom, which means you have a poor nutritional diet or a nutrition deficiency. There is a difference between the two, although the results could be the same. Your body produces 75% of its own cholesterol, it is used for arterial wall repair. It is also the building block of bile, and it helps move oxygen to starved parts of the body. It sounds like something the body truly needs.

The numbers are to scare you, because you don't know the language of numbers, therefore they are interpreted to you incorrectly. Honestly I am not sure if most doctors know the language although they are a secret society. This subject is an entire lecture, so let's just look at some natural ways of dealing with this issue: *Carrot & celery juice a 16 oz. glass once a day works well. Guggul and lecithin work to reduce cholesterol levels. Stay away from fried foods.*

Diabetes: Regardless of the type of diabetes, it is a pancreas problem, and an issue of providing enough energy for the body, through the break-down of carbohydrates. Type I is usually found in children and type II in adults. Type I not enough insulin, Type II enough insulin, but not absorbed by the receptors. For this formula to be effective, you will need the combination of minerals and vitamins: *vanadyl sulfate, chromium, bilberry, gynmena sylvestre, and bitter melon.*

Fibroid tumors: Afrakan women are highly affected by this disharmony. The muscle fiber of the uterus weakens and develops a bump like ballooning-out similar to a hemorrhoid or varicose vein. Inside the fibroid capsule, there can be rotten blood, trapped veins, arteries, cellular waste, and fluid pus. They tend to shrink during menopause due to decreased estrogen production. The stressed liver can not neutralize waste and therefore contribute to the growth of the fibroids. The size of the tumor is not nearly as important as the location. The formula: *Glutathione is used to help shrink tumors, Manganese improves health of uterus, Potassium excretes cellular waste. Herbs would be Shepard's Purse, Witch hazel, White Oak Bark, and Burdock. Also a product called "can X" (black salve) dissolves tumors.*

Prostate: This is part of urinary system as well as your reproductive system. The prostate inflames around the urethra and problems begin. Sometimes it is just simple inflammation, others times it is forms of cancer, but it all can be dealt with naturally. This is caused by poor nutrition and excessive sexual ejaculation. There is a spiritual understanding of having sex, so not to ejaculate all the time. A formula would consist of ; saw palmetto, buchu, horsetail, couch grass and maybe some pumpkin seed and echinacea. buchu, horsetail, couch grass, echinacea are also good for UTI's.

Varicose Veins: The arteries become hard, and inflexible. This is the secondary problem. The primary problem is the body can't excrete the toxins effectively. Hardening can be caused by absence of fluid. A formula: *Cat's claw, to remove the toxins, Hawthorn to help the heart pump, Comfrey, garlic, witch hazel, marigold, and garlic.*

HAZARDS OF ALLOPATHIC MEDICINES

Antibiotics: neomycin interferes with the absorption of iron. Tetracycline blocks the absorption of dietary minerals: conversely, taking minerals with an antibiotic will block the action of the antibiotic.

Anticonvulsants: can lower the level of copper and zinc.

Magnesium & aluminum antacids: deplete calcium, phosphate.

Arthritis medications, such as D-penicillamine (Cuprimine)—can reduce absorption of zinc, iron, and probably some other minerals.

Aspirin—can cause enough blood loss through the stomach over time to cause an iron deficiency; it can also cause potassium depletion.

Cholesterol—lowering drugs—can reduce the iron that the body stores.

Estrogen replacement therapy—can deplete magnesium

Laxatives reduce absorption of minerals.

Oral contraceptives—tend to increase levels of copper, which in excess can cause a decrease in blood levels of iron and zinc; they also reduce levels of magnesium and selenium.

Alcohol—depletes iron, selenium, zinc, and magnesium.

Another scenario: if you have an irregular heart beat and high blood pressure and your Dr. prescribes a diuretic which will deplete magnesium, zinc, and potassium. It will only make your urinate the minerals that your heart requires so it is adding to the problem it is supposed to be curing, so they will probably prescribed another drug for you.

THE WHOLE PERSON

We have discussed that the whole person consists of; spirit, mind and body. What that means is: if your body is sick so is your mind. So let's look at how emotions are connected to the body, so we can see that you must see the whole body, to see you. If you can't see the whole person, then you are looking at life from a linear point of view. Part of you cannot be well and the other part sick. Do not segment yourself, know your connection to the Neteru, to the hidden Creator of all things, Amen.

Emotions are truly a language that we use on a regular basis, but have very little understanding of. Babies have the best understanding, and then mothers since they have given birth to the babies. An education connects you to your kulture, and through your kulture all healing is defined. The Afrakan kulture is not spoken much of in the educational world when it comes to giving birth to these great understandings of life. But the truth is within the Afrakan kulture you will find the deepest truth to many of the sciences and arts. History has been distorted to fit the needs of the ones writing it, as Napoleon once said "history is nothing more than an agreed upon lie." In a Western movie where a writer was following the story of a gun fighter and found out the gun fighter was not the fighter thought he was, the writer said "when the legend becomes fact, write about the legend." We love stories, because that is what we are taught; we value the myth over the truth. This connection to the whole body is not Chinese based, Native American based, India based, but Afrakan based, and the other kultures founded their principles on that which they learned out of Afraka.

Emotions are created by the Creator, but yet many of us feel as if an emotion belongs to us, and we can hold on to it forever; haven't you witnessed how some people appear to be always angry, or some people appear to be too happy, or some are always sick. Emotions are designed to move, that is what the word E-motion means, they move in you. You use them and they move out, otherwise they could kill you. So as the good book says "the power is in the word", I am telling you that the power is in the *thought*.

People will claim to understand their emotions, but to know about motions is to know beta-motion, alpha-motion, etc. so if you don't know these things, then you don't know emotions, you just think you do, this satisfies your ego, so you appear to be smart, to yourself. A smart person must recognize their disharmonies, and learn so that they can be healthy, because this is what it is all about.

When people get *angry* it is going to affect the body. The anger creates stress, the adrenal glands have to work overtime, and the kidney is affected, as well as the pancreas, which produces the energy for the kidney. Women, who develop a history of bad relationships with men, will be candidates for breast cancer. Everyone else will be a candidate for Kidney problems.

Stress, will burn out your adrenal glands, which means you have used an abundant amount of energy, which requires the pancreas to produce the insulin for this, and from stress alone one can develop diabetes.

Fear, have you ever felt that scared feeling in your stomach, it creates a chemical reaction, and gives the energy to fight if necessary and there is nothing in the digestive system for it to act on, now you have stressed out the digestive system if you stay in this mode, fear can also get trapped behind your heart and that can be painful. Fear can increase fat to the hips, breast and prostate.

You are probably wondering how can *happy* be harmful to the body, The problem is understanding the emotions, none of them are bad until you become locked into them or they begin to dominate your life. So it is Ok to be happy, but one must learn to use the other emotions. It is Ok to be angry if anger is going to save your life. It is Ok to experience fear, because the body pumps up the energy for it. We just need to learn how to use them, move in, and move out, otherwise disharmonies will come into the body.

Hormones are one element of directing the emotions, the main three, Estrogen, Progesterone, and Testosterone.

Emotions are also associated with eating habits:

- Bready—feelings of insecurity, dissatisfaction
- Chewy—relieves stress, tension
- Creamy—comfort, and nurturing
- Crunchy—releases anxiety
- Salty—redirects anger
- Sweet—the need for love or to give it

Everything in life is connected. We must save ourselves.

When the laws of Nature are violated, we pay. One must work at being healthy today, because money is in "sickness" so sickness has to be promoted, marketed and advertised. Money is more valuable than life.

Illness is not natural!

THE BABY

We are raising our babies like adults instead of like babies; we want them to eat like us and act like us, how ignorant of us. A baby is trying to digest the world.

It takes approximately 8 years for a baby's digestion system to mature. So how much stress are you putting on the baby? Is a question that must be asked by all parents. This means that the Baby doesn't have the enzymes to break down food like an adult. Afrakan grandmothers and mothers would chew the food for the baby, then put it in the baby's mouth, the salvia in the adults mouth starts coding the food, and breaks it down to digestible size for the body, if a baby is swallowing chunks of food, the system is stressing, and the child will be scarred with some type of illness behind that action. The baby is growing up with un-digested food in their stomach.

We are seeking a strong and healthy child, which will be based on the child's' nutrition. Therefore the child should be eating soft foods, plenty of fruits, so that the child develops a taste for fruits to find it's sugars, plenty of vegetables to keep the system alkaline. If we teach the child the right habits, then the child will live according to those habits, and these habits come from us knowing our kulture.

A child is the closest thing to the spiritual world, and we are taking that away with our eating habits, and conversations. Kulture is everything, so we must ask the right questions. We are caring for children according to whom or maybe I should say according to what? The fruits and vegetables are the only foods that will guarantee the child receiving the required nutrients it needs to get on the path. If the child needs a snack then have some fruit, quit giving a child de-natured food. When you are trying to sustain and promote growth, you can't be healthy from dead food, and the child needs plenty of live food, so it can be healthy, mentally as well as physically. Almost every illness a child has is due to poor nutrition.

As valuable a life is, how can we continue to mistreat children according to our ignorance? We are killing them, then we say we love them. If we love them then let us be educated on how to provide optimal care for their health. A lot of this is based on myth vs. fact, know the fact, and quit listening to those damn myths.

If the mother isn't breast feeding, then almond milk is a good substitute during this period of time. Once the child is done with milk, during those breast feeding years, it not ever drink another glass of milk in its entire life. It is Ok to breast a child for 3 or 4 years.

Feed the child soft foods, that are easily digestible, if a food is hard for you to chew, why would you expect a child to chew it.

God(dess) didn't create cereal and milk. That is a horrible combination. When Dr. Kellogg created corn flakes, it was to be a natural nutritious meal, then someone said let's drink some milk with it. Myth: that man has always fed children cow's milk, fact: western world didn't start using cow's milk until the 1700's. Fact: after Louis created his pasteurizing processing for milk, he admitted that his approach was unhealthy, but the world had starting making money, so it was disregarded. 50 years ago a cow only produced about 2 quarts of milk. With the usage of today's hormones they are now producing up to 50 quarts a day. The milk is a poison for humans.

Fruits for breakfast, and a combination of vegetables for dinner. Try to keep the fruits and vegetables very diverse with your eating. One day you eat bananas and pears, the next day melons, the next day apples. The rawer the food the better, raw has its own enzymes so now the child's body doesn't have to do all the work, in trying to break the food down.

When meat is cooked, the enzymes are cooked out, and that is another horrible story that is taking place inside of the child's digestion system.

Remove your emotions, and follow Maat. If you have had your share of illnesses, why would you want your child to suffer through that, which means, if you want a different result then you must do something different.

America promotes what is called an anti-thyroid diet, which is harmful in so many ways, I can't list them all, but it throws the body out of rhythm, when out of rhythm, you are susceptible to all and any disease.

Many times new born babies will know what foods they like and don't like. Don't force feed the child that is you trying to make it like you. The study of pediatrics it isn't that hard. There are plenty of nutritional books and information available on what constitutes a good meal for a child. Any and all processed food is wrong for the child. If God(dess) didn't grow it, don't feed it, that is what you owe your child. Give the child a chance, Please!

VITAMINS

. . . And god said, "Behold, I have given you every herb bearing seed, which is upon the face of all the earth, and every tree, in the which is the fruit of a tree yielding seed, to you it shall be for meat . . . .

Genesis 1:29, 30.

Why is not the preacher teaching about a healthy body? You can not have a healthy body, and a sick mind, or a healthy mind and a sick body. If one is sick then you are sick. We are all familiar with the saying: *that you can't separate the mind and body . . .* We have forgotten how to think when it comes to ourselves, but we are quick to have an answer for what everyone else should be doing.

A mineral is a vitamin (vital mineral), a vitamin is a hormone, and a hormone is an enzyme. As the behavior changes so does the name, and the medical society keeps the community confused.

Vitamins come from the plants and vegetables, which validate that "mother earth" provides all we need to sustain ourselves from the ground, which is rich in minerals, and our edible life grows from it.

There are those who don't promote vitamins, because they believe it can be obtained from the food. Since the food is synthetic and poisoned, so we need help, through the supplements of vitamins and herbs. The environment has changed for the worse over the last thousand years. We live in a so-called advanced world, but that confuses me, because over the last 100 years we have created the most destruction to the world in world history. I guess the definition of advanced needs to be changed. We have more diseases today than yesterday, and the list continues to grow. The majority of the population is living a low quality life as far as health is concerned under the disguise that they are living a normal life.

Anything not in balance with Nature (neteru) is living an un-natural life, which by default is unhealthy. There is plenty of research that says, vitamin therapy has shown remarkable work in restoring the health of the sick.

Sometimes the answer is not in research. The spiritual essence of energy from people, animals or plants cannot be measured by research, no more than God can be defined by the intellect. Sometimes as healers we must simply listen to how the client feels, everyone should know how to be in-tune with their own bodies.

We believe in God, but we put our lives in the hands of Men, and for the most part ignorant men, because education is not the same as wisdom, and science does not define the spirit. In truth the more intellectual we become the further from God we drift. Our instincts have become weaker, and we have misjudged the truth. Any education that does not enhance you mentally and physically is not worth having and is segmented learning.

We need to return to the indigenous ways of our ancestors, the truth they left us, is still true today.

Unfortunately the Health industry is not in the health business, but in the business of economics, because there is no money in healthy people. As long you are sick the rich will get richer.

The RDA, which is *recommended dietary allowance*, is not necessarily accurate. It is designed for a person trying to maintain health, not a person who is trying to restore health, and this is where the natural healers should be consulted.

The bottom line is without vitamins; our bodies would quit functioning, is that enough to make us take this serious.

We will now look at various vitamins, and evaluate their formulas for restoring health and maintaining health.

Be aware, that all Vitamins have a family. This family isn't talked about, because that would be educating too much according to the medical society, although they aren't as brilliant as you may think. Here we will mention some of the families as needed. One of the simplest ways of making sure you are getting the whole family is look for "complex" on the label, or if you can convince your Doctor to give you a shot, they can administer high doses of vitamins, but they don't want to teach that, or you may try to fix yourself through vitamins. Nothing replaces eating nutritionally, with diversity.

INDIVIDUAL VITAMINS

As with herbs, vitamins have multiple purposes, so we will try to mention some of their primary functions, and the causes of deficiencies.

Vitamin A, is good for repairing tissues that have been traumatized through surgery or injury. It is good for smooth skin, helps with resistance to colds, it is also involved with sexual functioning. Oral contraceptives deplete Vitamin A and of course it is popular for eye health, without it the eyes will start to dry out, which leads to eye diseases.

We have mentioned how every part of the body is connected to each other, so let's review some examples: A heavy drinker, can have serious eye problems. The alcohol has a detrimental effect on the liver, which prevents the liver from storing Vitamin A, and mobilizing it, therefore without that Vitamin A, the eyes can't produce a substance called "visual purple" which is necessary for seeing at night. Glaucoma which is stiffness in the eye, an arthritis type problem, which comes from drying out, or lack of moisture, this occurs in the eye without enough Vitamin A.

If we are getting the vitamins from the food, why are these diseases on the rise?

A person with Crohns disease is holes in the intestines, if these holes are large enough, then vitamins and minerals fall through, and the person isn't absorbing the necessary nutrients. Vitamin A has shown to help bowel movements return to normal.

Vitamin A also helps build healthy teeth.

Vitamin A has been found to help patients with cancer treatment

Vitamin A has been found to be healthy for the circulatory system.

An entire chapter can be dedicated to these herbs, so the list doesn't stop here, but shares some useful information about the vitamin.

As the vitamin and herbs supply our bodies, keep in mind that different amounts are needed by different organs and systems in the body, and even though sometimes the amount may be very minute, but essential. I can't over emphasize the word **essential**.

Vitamin A will offer you some cushion through many of life's depressing environments.

Vitamin B, in this section we shall talk about the "family" of Vitamin B, because it is well known to the public, but don't forget that all vitamins have a family.

Each B vitamin has a specific function, but nutrients work in aid of each other, cooperatively, or shall I say in harmony with each other, so that they aid each other.

Earlier it was mentioned that: a mineral is a vitamin, a vitamin a hormone, a hormone an enzyme. B vitamins operate more like co-enzymes.

Vitamin B$_1$ which is thiamine, without thiamine the brain and nervous system would collapse. A deficiency of it shows symptoms of senility, and memory loss. Even though only small amounts are needed, it is essential. Japanese studies show that it strengthens the heart.

Diabetics usually have low levels of thiamine.

Chlorine destroys thiamine, so cooking in tap water is depleting foods that have thiamine, such as rice, so cook with distilled water.

Vitamin B$_2$ which is riboflavin can be host to many problems if a deficiency is occurring: (cataracts, fatigue, birth defects, and cancer) a pinkish colored tongue is a good indicator that you are receiving enough. If you have oily hair, lines radiating from your lips, frequent tearing of the eyes, any and all of these may improve with riboflavin.

Oral contraceptives and tranquilizers inhibit the absorption of this vitamin. B vitamins are water soluble; therefore you lose these vitamins, if you soak your vegetables in water before cooking them, or cooking your food too hot.

Riboflavin is essential in building healthy red blood cells.

Niacin a member of the B vitamin family which is essential to your brain otherwise thoughts become weak, and emotions shaky. There are other mental disturbances than can take place with a deficiency of niacin, such as; depression, irritability, memory loss, nervousness, apprehension, and the list goes on as if out of a neurotic diary.

Niacin restores the electrical charge in red blood cells as they are supplied to your brain and heart. When this electrical charge is lost, blood cells have a tendency to clump together blocking the flow through capillaries. Doctors have long known, that niacin helps to break up blood fats like cholesterol, which clog up arteries when oxidized, cholesterol becomes oxidized when a person has poor nutrition, therefore affecting the heart. So cholesterol is not the cause of clogged arteries or heart problems, poor nutrition is and Niacin may help, but it does not replace good nutrition.

Niacin has also shown to help improve pellagra, which is a skin disharmony.

Niacin can be found in whole grains, and in B-complex, Brewers yeast is a good source.

Vitamin B$_6$ is pyridoxine; it doesn't have the status of the other B vitamins, but can help prevent some side effects from prescription drugs, including oral contraceptives. It is now being used on hyperactive children, diabetes mellitus, infertility, and some others.

Inadequate B$_6$ may manifest itself as carpal tunnel syndrome; remember a syndrome is a series of symptoms. When one part of the body is affected, so is the whole system.

Over refined cooked diets contribute to the deficiency of this vitamin.

With all the environmental factors the RDA is far too low, especially when one of these diseases has occurred. When the symptom has shown itself on the outside of your body, it has already manifested on the inside of the body, so we need healing and that goes beyond recommended dosages.

B$_6$ has proven its self effective against the "Chinese restaurant syndrome", which is after eating a heavy spiced meal with MSG, one gets a headache, feverish flush, and feeling of being uneasy.

B$_6$ helps with the prevention of kidney stones, carpal tunnel syndrome, and helps to keep blood clots away.

Vitamin B$_{12}$ is very effective against various nerve disorders, allowing us to quit saying things such as "too many things on my mind to remember" that is not an excuse, that is a cop-out. Or its Monday morning so I am tired. Instead of a cup of coffee, let's try boosting our B$_{12}$ intake and you might be surprised.

The sources are rare, Drs. can give you an injection, the body does produce its own in small amounts, it can also be obtained from Brewers Yeast, B-complex, spring water, and in animals, but I am not an advocate of eating animal products.

This vitamin has reversed many physical disharmonies. The body stores this vitamin, and you only need small amounts, but the acid stress on the body is reducing it, and it is not being replenished through our eating habits.

Most test for deficiencies of this vitamin are unreliable. The RDA is 3 micrograms daily.

Folate is folic acid and is essential to the body in a variety of ways, such maintaining the integrity of the blood and nerves. It helps prevent senility, because it is dominate in the spinal fluid. It has shown to improve the mood of people. Folate allows the memories of genes to be passed on to other genes, in birth.

Folate is a sensitive nutrient, highly found in vegetables, if you boil your vegetables you need to drink the water. Vitamin C is also lost in the boiling of vegetables, therefore drinking the water you will recover some other nutrients beside the Folate

Medical research says this is the most deficient vitamin in man.

Antibiotics and pain killers are two of the most abused drugs in the world, and antibiotics deplete Folate. Folate is manufactured in the intestinal tract, which is filled with plague by most unhealthy eaters, therefore nutrients aren't absorbed fully and the B vitamin manufacturing process is compromised. The antibiotics are destroying the B vitamins while it is in the intestines.

Hopefully we can get a picture of how each part of the body is affected by the next. We are whole people.

Pantothenate, an anti-stress B vitamin. Actually it turns into a co-enzyme, co-enzyme A or CoA. CoA is vital to the health of the adrenal glands, and the production of its hormones. Remember earlier, we mentioned that a vitamin is a hormone, a hormone is an enzyme, the name changes when the behavior changes. It is also good against radiation, and stress.

Pantos is the Greek word for everywhere, and Pantothenate is everywhere, you can find it in almost all foods. Not in the frozen section but fresh foods.

There is no RDA for this vitamin.

PABA is a B vitamin that protects you against UVB wavelengths of the sun

Biotin is under a lot of research, it is needed to maintain the functioning of certain enzymes, and very hard to test for a deficiency.

Choline is being studied for improving memory.

Vitamin B_{15} the last of the B vitamins we will discuss. It has been known to help with heart disease, diabetes, schizophrenia, alcoholism and asthma.

Vitamin C is a water soluble vitamin that performs numerous healing actions. Sometimes we know it as ascorbic acid, which is only a member of the C vitamin family. Vitamin C is probably the Noble prize winner of the vitamins. The body doesn't store this vitamin; therefore an adequate amount needs to be consumed each day.

By increasing the dosage for various disharmonies, vitamin C has been found to reverse the ill effects.

Vitamin C allows the body to absorb iron.

It neutralizes chlorine which is in tap water, chlorine destroys red blood cells.

Heat stress burns up vitamin C, and vitamin C helps rid heat rash.

Vitamin C taken daily in large enough doses, helps to prevent a host of disharmonies. Dosages have to be regulated on the type of disharmony, and the lifestyle of the individual to be accurate, this should be done with the consultation of a professional who knows vitamins, standardized numbers work for standard people. I have yet to figure out what a standard person is.

Vitamin C also helps with cholesterol levels by enhancing the production of HDL cholesterol; it also promotes the transporting of cholesterol to the bile acids so it can be excreted.

Research has shown that it may inhibit the growth of cancerous cells. It has reversed tumor growths.

Vitamin C (ascorbic acid) has shown to aid in heroin addictions, in a unique healthy process. Bioflavonoids are essential for the absorption of ascorbic acid, Bioflavonoids are found in many berry type fruits. So this is a step in changing lifestyle, because the eating habits have to be changed, we have already shown a variety of healthy things that happen to the body when nutritional food is eaten, and supplemented by herbs and vitamins.

Vitamin C is truly essential to optimal health, and needs to be taken daily. It is a key element in optimal health. Fruit bioflavonoids are known as citrus bioflavonoids, which are helpful with the repair of capillaries.

Heavy nose bleeding can be due to weak capillaries. The hospital will try to burn them close to stop the bleeding, but citrus flavonoids will help repair them naturally so you won't have that problem anymore.

The discussion of Vitamin C is almost endless, but you can never go wrong by trying a Vitamin C therapy program for any disharmony, although it is always recommended that you consult with a health professional.

Vitamin D a vitamin sometimes referred to as a hormone more than a vitamin. We have all heard the commercials, "drink milk, it builds strong bones". The truth is it allows for strong bones to be built. Vitamin D allows calcium to be absorbed, which is key in making the bone strong. The vitamin D that is added to milk is D_2 which is the wrong vitamin D for bone growth, once the milk is pasteurized all nutrients are lost, so they add some synthetic junk back into it.

Vitamin D is also known as the "sunshine vitamin" the energy of the sun allows the skin to manufacture vitamin D, so living in cold weather places, reduces that ability.

Once again we see how elements are connected, Vitamin D is crucial in the metabolism of calcium, so if your Vitamin D levels are down, then you are probably suffering from a calcium deficiency as well.

Inside the bones are where white blood cells are created, which fight off foreign invaders in the body. So strong bones not only support the physical body, but the internal body in having an effective immune system.

The winter effect is known as SAD (seasonal affective disorder) which has contributed to depression. In one state where it rains a lot, the suicide rate is high; therefore we must look at the sun as a nutrient to the body. Afrakan people require two hours of sunlight a day. The high melanin count requires high energy, other groups can get away with 30-45 minutes a day.

Research is now investigating if there is a link between colon cancer and Vitamin D. Keeping in mind that it might not directly be the Vitamin D, but the calcium.

Vitamin E is best known for its effect on the blood, sometimes used as a blood thinner for people with high blood pressure therefore making it a good vitamin for circulation. Also known to help protect the eyes.

Vitamin E is as versatile as Vitamin C, but it is fat soluble, meaning that the body stores it.

Vitamin E, helps promote a strong heart, protects cell membranes, lowers cholesterol, it helps heal skin, for burns and abrasions it can be taken orally, and locally. It helps with cold sores, which are forms of herpes. The free radicals that we breathe, Vitamin E helps to neutralize them.

It is also being used on children with cystic fibrosis.

Different types of nuts are good sources of Vitamin E, such as almonds, pecans, hazelnuts, sunflower seeds, to list a few sources.

Vitamin K is a vitamin given little attention, but it is as crucial as the others. We know that it is important in the coagulation of blood, and bleeding occurs inside of the body as well as on the outside that which you see, and that which you don't see. It is now believed critical in bone maintenance.

There is no one good source, it is plentiful in nature.

We have now gone through the list vitamins and read about their importance. As we did with the herbs we shall explore some formulas using vitamins, but I will also show what herbs can be added to some of the formulas.

FYI: all products are not equal, just because brand A says Vitamin C, does not mean it is of the same quality as brand B. Unfortunately we must do our research on the companies, and many times we will be choosing between the worse of two evils, and that is the world we live in.

Organic is always better than conventional, if one is trying to eat healthier.

Now that the FDA has approved the sale of cloned meat, people have no idea what they are eating.

We live in a time when the people must become aware of their own health, if they are to be healthy, not just your physical body, but your mental well being, they are connected, because the brain is so easy to trick, we have forgotten how to assess ourselves. Before we pray for others, we need to pray for our individual selves.

Our education has been more myth than fact; we live in a world of theories.

Ask yourself the real definition of an insane mind, then ask yourself could you possibly be insane. I ask you a question: how much education have you had about the brain?

If you want to quit being a victim, then quit creating it.

Do not allow your emotion to make the decision. In most cases to find the truth you must be willing to discover your own dark secrets.

In understanding your Kulture, that will take you a long way in having good health, mentally and physically.

Disharmonies and Formulas with Vitamins

The list of disharmonies is to exhaustive to list them all, so I shall share some common ones, that most people are familiar with.

Acne: the skin is dependant upon vitamin A, Vitamin A levels are depended upon Zinc. I would recommend vitamin A & Zinc. Possibly some vitamin E as well.
Herbs: comfrey, burdock, cleavers,

Cancer: Vitamin C & B$_{12}$ of course intravenously would be the way to go, 1 part B12, 2 parts C. If taking tablets, it would take large doses.(*Drs. Have a purer version of vitamins that they can write a prescription for.*). a recommended formula; folic acid, selenium, B$_{12}$, vitamin e, beta-carotene.
Herbs: myrrh, astragalus, msm, dandelion, echinacea, red clover, goldenseal.

Colds: large does of Vitamin C, as much as 6,000 mg a day, and Zinc.
Herbs: garlic, slippery elm, echinacea, goldenseal, rose hips.

Cramps: Vitamin E has shown to be effective with muscular cramps.
Herbs: chamomile, white willow, blue cohosh, thyme, valerian.

Hair loss: The B vitamin family, especially Pantothenate (helps to thicken hair), Folate and B$_6$.
Herbs: burdock, chaparral, nettle, horsetail, rosemary.

Hay fever (allergies): Vitamin C aided by citrus bioflavonoids.
Herbs: burdock, mullein, astragalus, marshmallow root.

Heart Disease: Vitamin C, E, and niacin as well as some flax seed.
Herbs: cramp bark, hawthorn, cinchona, lily of the valley

Skin Disharmonies: large does of Vitamin A, Vitamin E, and Zinc.
Herbs: cleavers, burdock, comfrey, nettle, red clover.

HOLISTIC LIFE

The combining of herbs, minerals and vitamins is the complete and true utilization of nature. If God didn't create it, then it ain't natural, and it doesn't belong with nature.

Good health does not exist with synthetic products, so doctors know they really can't recommend a change in diet, because most of the food has **no** nutritional value and they are not in the nutrition business, their understanding of Natural healing is almost none existent and even less practiced. The food has been the cause of many disharmonies. The combination of foods is very important as well. The wrong combinations will result in un-digested food, which eventually becomes toxic.

When your lifestyle is based upon one from another kulture, you can only be as healthy as those of that kulture. Which by default still makes you sick, not just physically, but mentally as well. Our emotions are what keep people trapped in some of these insane decisions we make about our well-being, and education has made us ignorant of it.

Aids and Cancer are no longer diseases, but business. We must know how to find our good health.

We need the correct food, the correct music, the correct Gods(desses), the correct environment to be healthy. We are as much a part of Nature as it is of us. We destroy it, and that is self destruction.

You are a whole person, therefore you can't be measured by a standard, because there is no standard person. We are designed to have different lifestyles, because our purposes in life are different. Diversity is nature, and so must our skills and talents, so we live differently, but still it must be in harmony. This harmony is must be our balance with Nature as well as with our community or village.

We must be willing to re-educate, while finding that which is appropriate knowledge for our existence to be all it can be, we are a long way from what it was designed to be.

Spirit, mind and body equals the whole person.

BLOOD

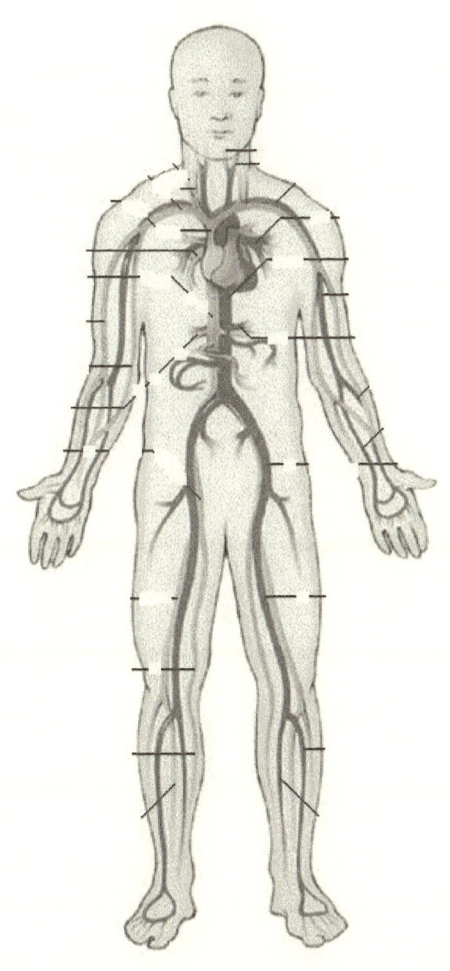

Blood Cleansing	*Circulatory stimulation*	*Normalizing*
burdock root	ginkgo biloba	dandelion
pau d' arco	hawthorn	alfalfa
sarsaparilla	ginger root	kelp
licorice root	blessed thistle	yellow dock
red clover	motherwort	marshmallow

BONES

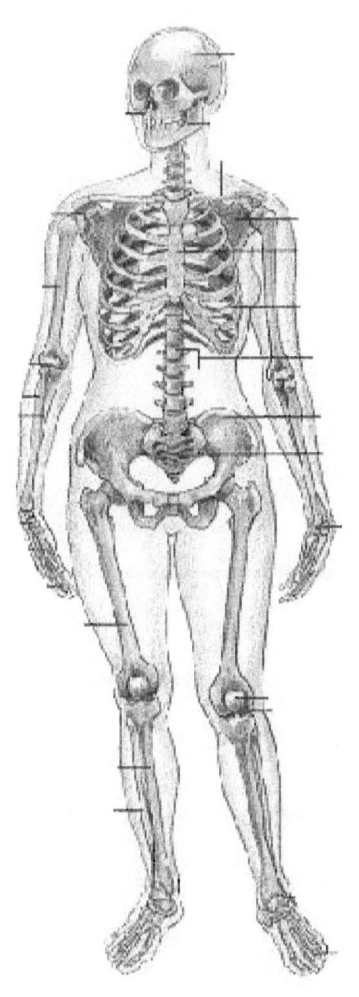

Bone strength
msm
white oak bark
comfrey
glucosamine
black cohosh

Healing broken bones
horsetail
nettles
golden seal
chlorella
sea vegetables

MUSCLES

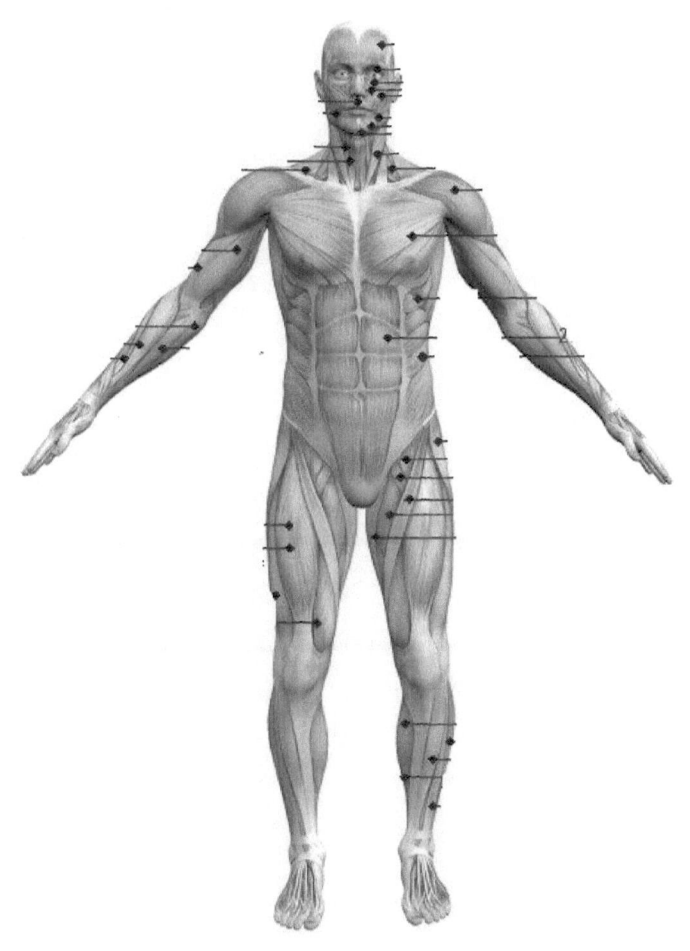

Muscle tone
bee pollen
ginger root
sarsaparilla root
barley grass
licorice root
sea vegetables

NERVES

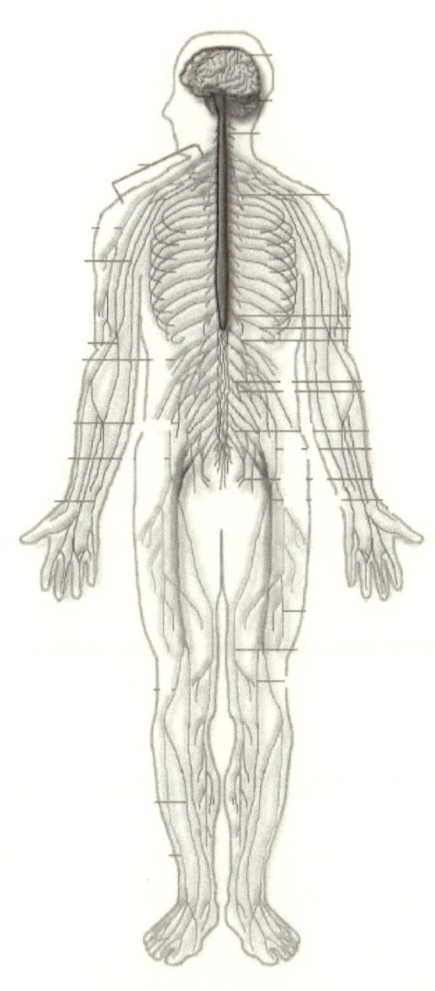

scullcap
lady slipper
rosemary
valerian
chamomile
kava kava
lobelia

Heart

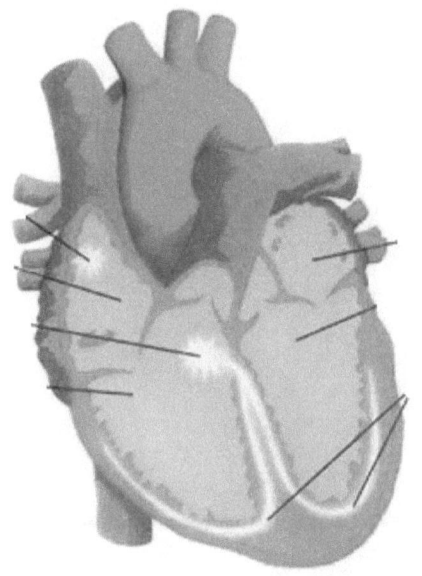

Weak heart
motherwort
hawthorn
lime blossom
lily of the valley
ginger

High blood pressure
cramp bark
motherwort
mistletoe
yarrow
bilberry

RESPIRATORY SYSTEM

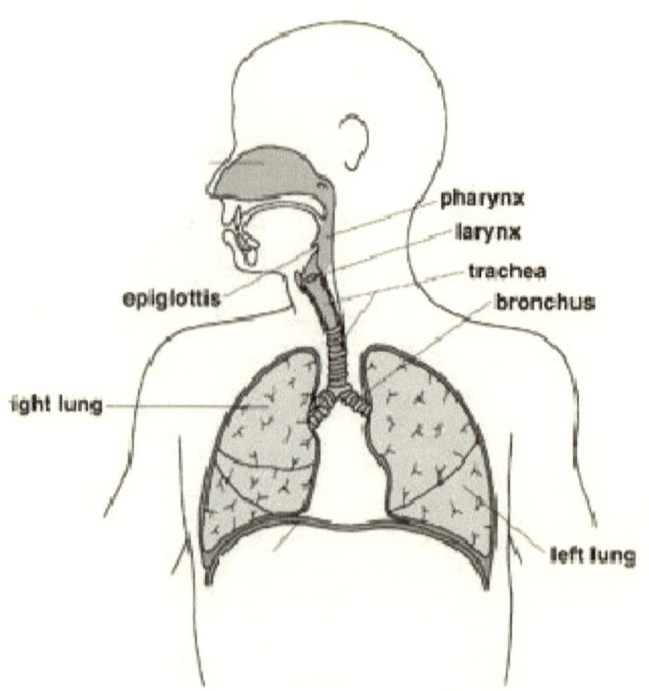

pharynx
larynx
trachea
bronchus
epiglottis
right lung
left lung

Mullein
Ephedra
pleurisy root
fenugreek
lobelia
marshmallow

Liver, gallbladder, & spleen

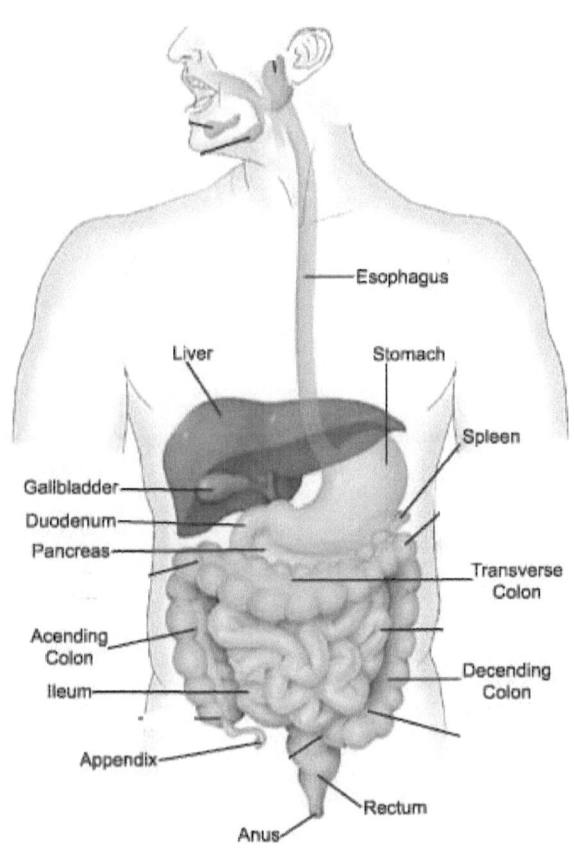

- Esophagus
- Liver
- Stomach
- Spleen
- Gallbladder
- Duodenum
- Pancreas
- Transverse Colon
- Acending Colon
- Decending Colon
- Ileum
- Appendix
- Rectum
- Anus

Liver
dandelion
milk thistle
yellow dock
alfalfa
sea vegetables

Gallbladder
dandelion
marshmallow
golden seal
gotu kola
astragalus

Spleen
siberian ginsing
licorice root
burdock
oregon grape
dandelion

KIDNEY

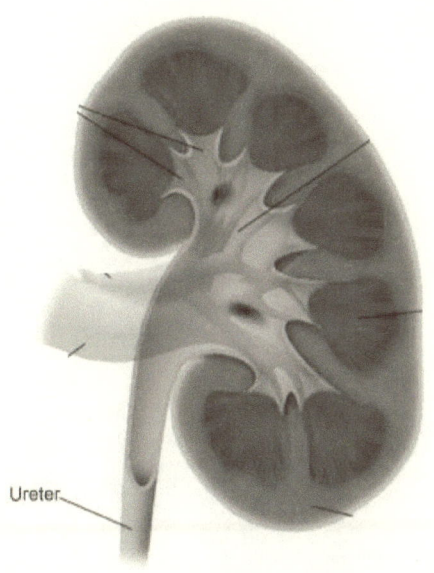

Ureter

dandelion
poke root
parsley
cornsilk
nettles
juniper berry
green tea
alfalfa

DIGESTION SYSTEM

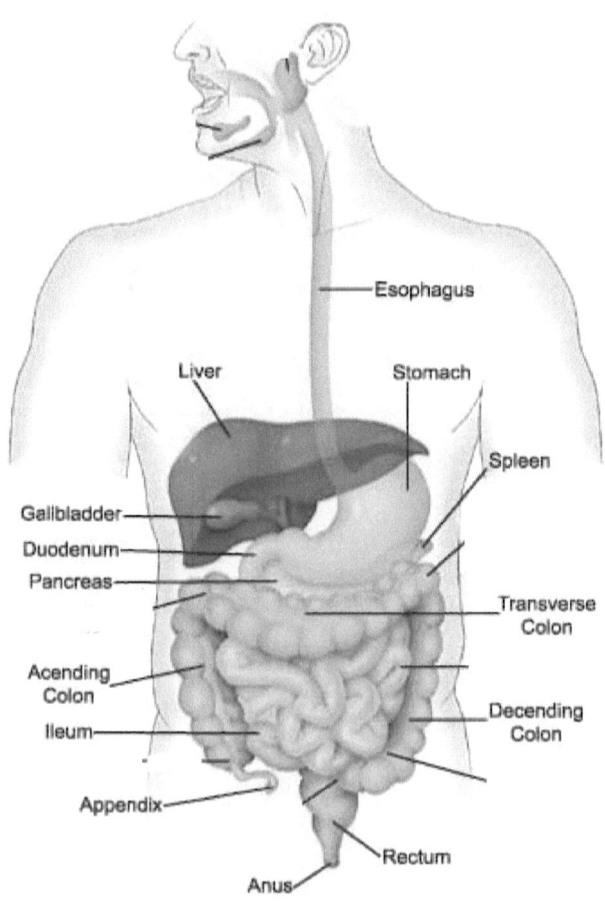

Esophagus

Liver

Stomach

Spleen

Gallbladder

Duodenum

Pancreas

Transverse Colon

Acending Colon

Decending Colon

Ileum

Appendix

Rectum

Anus

Garlic
fennel seed
sea vegetables
alfalfa
catnip
slippery elm
Elimination: cascara sagrada, comfrey, flaxseed, chlorophyll

Skin
comfrey
burdock
evening primrose
zinc

Hair
rosemary
sage
jojoba oil
Growth: horsetail, cayenne, nettles

Vision
eyebright
bilberry
calendula
burdock root

Brain
ginkgo biloba
chlorella
royal jelly
sage

GLANDS

Adrenal glands
royal jelly
licorice root
astragalus
sarsaparilla root

Pituitary gland
damiana
dong quai
burdock
alfalfa

Lymph
chaparral
echinacea
barberry bark
green tea

Pancreas
juniper berries
licorice root
bilberry
bittermelon

Ovaries
dong quai root
damiana
wild yam root
uva ursi

Thymus gland
bee pollen
echinacea
fenugreek
barley grass

Thyroid
sea vegetables
chlorella
lobelia
parsley

Testes
panax ginseng
dandelion
licorice root
damiana

I hope you have enjoyed this journey about your own health. The medicine of today dictates that we learn how to heal ourselves and do it in harmony with Nature, as the Creator designed it to be!

I cannot over emphasize the following: We must begin to think again, what we call thoughts are expressions of emotions without knowledge, because the ego has tricked the brain into not recognizing the difference. We have substituted science knowledge for spiritual knowledge, while we watch the world get worse and still we haven't figured out how we must change ourselves. We have used these tired, self-serving thoughts of ours to keep us feeling good for so long, that we now call the truth a lie. The improper nutrition consumed has the ability to throw ones' thoughts off the square, which is out of balance with life itself. As if an altered life is being lived as the real one, the real being the one that balances with the laws of Nature, which keeps life healthy and vibrant and very spiritually connected.

You cannot have good health from dead products and that's the bottom line. Knowing this, who would continue to do such a thing except for an insane mind. Are you starting to see the picture? Get away from those TV definitions of life, and find the real meanings and you will find your true health. Good health must include spirit, mind and body. the whole person needs to have whole health, and then one is on the square. If the body is sick so is the mind, it is probably the sick thoughts that created the sick behaviors which made the body sick. Sick thoughts are thoughts which keep you from developing into your greatness, and your greatness must be of benefit to others as well as yourself.

Health is a birthright which being stolen, through the food industries, pharmaceutical companies, hospitals, and all their affiliates. the freedom of choice is being taken away, and when people are ignorant of it, is easy to do. It is time for our greatness to be expressed. Knowledge is nothing without its application, so knowledge is not power, but the usage of knowledge is. We must use ours. *Quit being read to and read for*, reclaim your health, which is your greatest asset, demand that it be respected as such.

This list of herbs shared is only partial, and doesn't show exact combinations, it designed to share some recommended ideas, as well as some general understanding of how the earth provides for us.

For any type of illness, I recommend you consult your Health care provider.

SINGLE HERBS

Aloe (**Afraka**)—Constipation

Alum root—Astringent for wrinkles, diarrhea

Arnica—external use for pain, inflammation

Bilberry—eye problems, Vitamin C, diabetes

Black Cohosh—female estrogen hormone source

Bladderwrack—weight loss, thyroid, and kidney problems

Buchu—kidney, urinary pain, prostate irritation

Burdock—blood cleanser, liver, carry dead cells out to the body

Butcher's Broom—healthy cell growth, cleans veins, hemorrhoids

Calendula—stop bleeding

Capsicum (cayenne)—circulation, stops unnatural bleeding

Cascara Sagrada—encourages bile flow

Cat's Claw—anti-inflammatory

Catnip—Nerves, helps with sleep, expels gas

Chamonmile—restlessness

Chaste Tree Berry—fibroid tumors

Chickweed—blood cleanser, skin

Comfrey—constipation

Cornsilk—Kidney, urinary tract, rich in vitamin K

Damiana—sexual stimulant for both sexes, hot flashes

Dandelion root—liver cleanser and skin disorders, diuretic

Dandelion leaf—vitamin A, potassium

Devil's claw—deteriorating bones, arthritis

Dong Quai—regulates estrogen levels, for females

Echinacea—blood cleanser, antibiotic

Ephedra—Stimulant, adrenaline

Eyebright—most eye problems

Fennel—curbs appetite, good for excess stomach acid

Fenugreek—dissolves cholesterol

Feverfew—migraine headaches, and fevers

Flax—good for digestion

Fo-ti—circulation

Garlic—cleanser, antibiotic

Ginger—diaphoretic, dyspeptic, abnormal blood clotting, high blood pressure

Ginkgo Biloba—improves circulation to the brain

Golden Seal—tonic, infections

Grape Seed—anti-oxidant

Hawthorn—supports the heart

Horny goat weed—sexual appetite, reproductive system

Hops—calm nerves

Horehound—sore throat with coughs

Inkberry (Pokeroot)—dissolves cancers and tumors

Irish Moss—essential minerals, rebuilds connective tissue

Juniper Berries—Kidneys, gout & rheumatic discomfort

Licorice Root (DGL)—low blood sugar, natural cortisone, ulcers

Marshmallow—Kidneys

Milk Thistle—Liver

Mullein—Lungs

Milkweed—venereal disease, chest and abdominal complaints

Parsley—excellent source of iron, diuretic

Psyllium Seed Husk—adds bulk to the bowels, lubricates digestion

Pumpkin Seed—prostate, important for zinc absorption

Sassafras—thins the thick blood, use on poison ivy

Saw Palmetto—reproductive system, for men, enlarges breast in women

Scullcap—mild headaches, calms

Senna—bowel cleaner, magnesium (do not use often)

Shepard's purse—fibroids, hemorrhoids

Slippery Elm—Nutrient, healer, sore throat due to cold

Spirulina—protein and mineral source

Strawberries—good for brushing teeth (leaf for nite sweats)

Sunflower—vitamin D

Uva Ursi—Kidneys, bladder, diuretic

Valerian root—sleep, calms

White Clove—Sex organs

White Oak Bark—varicose veins, Hemorrhoids

Wild Lettuce—calms nerves

Wild Yam (black willow)—drains sinus, progesterone

Willow—natural aspirin

Yerba Santa—drains fluids from lungs

Yokum—Afrakan aphrodisiac, hot flashes

Please keep in mind all formulas are considered as recommendations. For any illness or disharmony it is highly recommended and advised that you consult your health provider before trying any formulas or recommendations.

No formula is guaranteed, but the research done on the various herbs and vitamins are sound and well documented.

For Health workshops or classes by Dr. Amen-Sebek contact:
Hotep Health (513) 652-5515

www.ingramcontent.com/pod-product-compliance
Lightning Source LLC
Chambersburg PA
CBHW020358290526
45785CB00005B/2341